Chair Yoga For Weight Loss:

Fast and Healthy Belly Fat Loss in 15 minutes with Gentle Exercises - Designed for Seniors over 60

Christoph Hermann

Disclaimer:

The information provided in this book is for educational and informational purposes only. The content is not intended to be a substitute for professional medical advice, diagnosis, or treatment. Always seek the advice of your physician or qualified healthcare provider with any questions you may have regarding a medical condition or the suitability of chair yoga exercises for your individual needs.

The author and publisher of this book make no representations or warranties, express or implied, regarding the accuracy, completeness, or effectiveness of the information provided. The author and publisher shall not be liable for any direct, indirect, consequential, or incidental damages arising out of the use or misuse of the information contained in this book.

Participation in chair yoga exercises carries inherent risks, and individuals should use caution and common sense when engaging in physical activity. It is important to listen to your body, respect your physical limitations, and seek guidance from qualified professionals if you experience any pain or discomfort during exercise.

By using this book, you acknowledge and agree to assume full responsibility for your own health and well-being. You understand that the author and publisher are not responsible for any injury, loss, or damage that may result from following the exercises or information provided herein.

Contents

Chapter 1

Introduction

Welcome to **"Chair Yoga for Weight Loss: Fast and Healthy Belly Fat Loss in 15 minutes with Gentle Exercises - Designed for Seniors over 60"**! In these pages, you'll discover the transformative power of chair yoga and how it can enrich the lives of seniors in ways they never imagined.

Picture this: a group of seniors, ranging from sprightly 60-year-olds to wise 90-year-olds, gathered in a community center. They sit comfortably in chairs, their eyes twinkling with anticipation as they embark on their weekly chair yoga session. As the gentle music fills the room, they begin to move, flowing gracefully through each pose, breathing deeply, and finding peace in the present moment.

But what's the secret behind this seemingly simple practice? Why is chair yoga so important for seniors over 60?

The truth is, as we age, our bodies change. We may not move as freely as we once did, and daily activities that were once effortless can become challenging. This is where chair yoga steps in as a game-changer. It offers a gentle yet effective way for seniors to improve their flexibility, strength, balance, and overall well-being—all from the comfort of a chair.

Now, let me share a heartwarming story with you. It's about my own grandparents and the countless older adults I've had the privilege of working with over the years. Like many seniors, they faced the inevitable challenges that come with aging—stiff joints, reduced mobility, and sometimes, feelings of isolation.

But through the practice of chair yoga, they discovered a new lease on life. With each session, they became more flexible, more resilient, and more connected to themselves and each other. They laughed, they stretched, and they found joy in movement once again.

I remember one particular moment when my grandmother, who had struggled with chronic pain for years, told me with tears in her eyes, ***"I feel alive again."*** It was a powerful reminder of the profound impact that chair yoga can have, not just on the body, but on the spirit as well.

And so, dear reader, as you embark on this journey through "Chair Yoga for Weight Loss: Fast and Healthy Belly Fat Loss in 15 minutes with Gentle Exercises - Designed for Seniors over 60," know that you are not alone. Within these pages, you'll find the tools, the guidance, and the inspiration you need to live a healthy, fit, and fulfilling lifestyle, no matter your age or ability. So grab a chair, take a deep breath, and let's begin this transformative journey together.

Chapter 2

Benefits Of Chair Yoga For Seniors

1. Improved Flexibility:

Flexibility is a crucial aspect of maintaining physical health and vitality, especially as we grow older. It involves the ability of our muscles and joints to move through their entire range of motion, which allows us to move without difficulty in our daily activities. Chair yoga is a gentle yet powerful way for seniors to improve their flexibility, which can offer numerous benefits that can significantly enhance their quality of life.

Having improved flexibility means you have increased freedom of movement and agility. Seniors who regularly practice chair yoga find that simple tasks, such as reaching for objects on high shelves, bending down to tie shoelaces, or getting in and out of chairs, become more comfortable and easier. This newfound ease of movement allows seniors to be more independent, which builds self-confidence, empowering them to navigate their daily lives with grace and efficiency.

Additionally, flexibility is crucial in maintaining joint health and preventing musculoskeletal problems commonly associated with aging. By integrating gentle stretching exercises into their routine, seniors can reduce stiffness and tension in their muscles and joints, which reduces the risk of chronic conditions like arthritis and enhances overall joint mobility. Moreover, improved flexibility encourages better posture since it allows muscles to maintain proper alignment, reducing strain and discomfort, which can lead to better spinal support.

Aside from the physical benefits, chair yoga's enhanced flexibility contributes to mental and emotional well-being. Many seniors feel a sense of liberation and vitality as they release tension and stiffness from their bodies. This newfound physical freedom is often accompanied by a profound sense of relaxation and calm, as the gentle, mindful movements of chair yoga promote a state of inner peace and tranquility.

Moreover, flexibility is a significant component of fall prevention, which is a crucial concern for seniors. By enhancing balance, coordination, and flexibility through chair yoga, seniors can significantly reduce their risk of falls and related injuries, maintaining their safety and independence for years to come.

In essence, the benefits of improved flexibility through chair yoga go beyond physical health. They include mental, emotional, and social well-being, enriching the lives of seniors in profound and transformative ways. Through regular practice, seniors can reclaim their mobility, vitality, and zest for life, embracing the golden years with grace, resilience, and joy.

2. Increased Strength:

Strength is a fundamental aspect of mobility, independence, and vitality, particularly among the elderly population. Chair yoga is a gentle yet effective practice that can also help seniors build strength, enabling them to overcome physical challenges and lead their lives with confidence and resilience.

One of the most notable benefits of chair yoga is the improvement of functional movement. Seniors who practice chair yoga engage in gentle yet effective strength-building poses and exercises that gradually strengthen their muscles, leading to enhanced efficiency and ease of performing daily tasks. This translates to greater independence and self-reliance in carrying out everyday activities such as lifting groceries, getting up from a seated position, or climbing stairs.

Similarly, chair yoga is also capable of helping seniors maintain appropriate posture and alignment, lowering their chance of developing common physical ailments like back pain and postural imbalances. Stronger muscles give better support for the spine and joints, reducing strain and discomfort while also improving general spinal health.

Chair yoga can be remarkably beneficial for seniors. Along with improving flexibility, it also helps increase strength, particularly in the core and lower body. This increased strength can greatly contribute to better balance and stability, which is essential for preventing falls among seniors. By strengthening the muscles that support the body, chair yoga can help seniors maintain coordination and balance, reducing the risk of falls and injuries. This newfound stability can instill a sense of confidence and security, empowering seniors to navigate their surroundings with greater ease and assurance.

Furthermore, building strength through chair yoga offers numerous benefits for overall health and well-being. Strength training has been shown to support healthy bone density, reducing the risk of osteoporosis and fractures, which is a common concern for seniors. Additionally, strength-building exercises can help seniors manage chronic conditions such as arthritis, by improving joint stability and reducing pain and inflammation.

Beyond the physical benefits, increased strength fosters a sense of empowerment and vitality in seniors. As they feel their muscles grow stronger and more resilient, many seniors report a renewed sense of energy and zest for life. This newfound strength extends beyond the physical realm, empowering seniors to tackle new challenges, pursue their passions, and live life to the fullest.

In essence, the benefits of increased strength through chair yoga are manifold, encompassing physical, emotional, and psychological well-being. Regular practice of chair yoga can help seniors cultivate strength, resilience, and vitality, enabling them to age gracefully and live their lives with confidence, purpose, and joy.

3. **Enhanced Balance:**

Maintaining a good balance is essential for people of all ages, but it becomes even more critical as we grow older. Chair yoga is a safe and effective way for seniors to improve their balance, which can help them move around with confidence and independence.

One of the most significant benefits of practicing chair yoga is the reduction of the risk of falls, which can cause severe injuries and affect seniors' ability to take care of themselves. By practicing various poses and exercises, seniors can strengthen the muscles that support their balance, improve their awareness of body position, and enhance their coordination, which promotes stability and reduces the risk of falls.

Improved balance through chair yoga can also help seniors feel more confident and self-assured, leading to more social interactions and a more fulfilling life. Moreover, better balance can contribute to better posture and alignment, reducing discomfort and pain in the spine and the joints. It also supports healthy circulation and cardiovascular function, which is beneficial for overall physical health and well-being.

Beyond physical benefits, chair yoga also incorporates mindfulness practices and breathwork techniques that promote mental focus and concentration. This can help seniors maintain balance in all aspects of life, not just physical balance on the yoga mat.

In summary, chair yoga is an excellent way for seniors to improve their balance, which can help them feel more confident, independent, and healthier in all areas of life. With regular practice, seniors can cultivate balance in their body, mind, and spirit, enabling them to age gracefully and enjoy life to the fullest.

4. Joint Health:

Maintaining good joint health is incredibly important, especially as we age and that's why chair yoga can be such a great option for seniors.

Another great benefit of chair yoga is that it can help lubricate the joints and promote synovial fluid production, which can help minimize discomfort and reduce the risk of inflammation. Additionally, chair yoga can help improve joint stability and balance, which can be especially important for preventing falls and maintaining independence.

One of the best things about chair yoga is that it's a low-impact form of exercise, which means that it's gentle on the joints. This makes it a great choice for seniors with arthritis or other joint-related conditions. Overall, chair yoga offers a holistic approach to improving joint health and promoting flexibility, stability, and comfort in daily life.

5. Stress Reduction:

Stress is an inevitable part of life, but as we age, managing stress becomes increasingly important for overall health and well-being. Chair yoga offers seniors a gentle yet powerful tool for stress reduction, providing a sanctuary of calm amidst life's challenges.

One of the most significant benefits of chair yoga for stress reduction is its emphasis on deep breathing and mindfulness practices. Through guided breathing exercises and mindful movement, seniors can cultivate a sense of inner peace and relaxation, activating the body's natural relaxation response and counteracting the effects of stress.

Moreover, chair yoga encourages seniors to be present in the moment, focusing their attention on the sensations of their breath and the gentle movements of their body. This mindfulness practice helps seniors let go of worries about the past or future, allowing them to experience a sense of peace and contentment in the present moment.

Additionally, chair yoga promotes physical relaxation by releasing tension and tightness in the body. Gentle stretching exercises and restorative poses help to soothe tired muscles and alleviate physical discomfort, creating a sensation of relaxation and ease throughout the body.

Furthermore, chair yoga offers seniors a safe and supportive environment to explore and release emotions. Through gentle movement and breathwork, seniors can release pent-up stress and tension stored in the body, fostering emotional well-being and resilience.

Moreover, chair yoga can have profound benefits for mental and emotional health, reducing symptoms of anxiety, depression, and insomnia—all of which are common concerns for seniors. By promoting relaxation and inner calm, chair yoga empowers seniors to navigate life's challenges with greater ease and resilience.

In essence, chair yoga offers seniors a holistic approach to stress reduction, addressing the interconnectedness of mind, body, and spirit. Through regular practice, seniors can experience the profound benefits of reduced stress, including improved mood, better sleep, and enhanced overall well-being.

6. Improved Posture:

Posture is an important factor for overall health and well-being, particularly for seniors. Chair yoga is an effective method for improving posture, promoting spinal alignment, and enhancing core strength. The focus of chair yoga poses is on spinal alignment, which helps reduce strain on the back and neck, promoting a tall, upright posture. Through regular practice, seniors can notice improvements in their posture, with shoulders back, chest open, and spine elongated. Chair yoga also strengthens the muscles that support good posture, particularly the core muscles, which are essential for maintaining proper alignment and posture. Additionally, chair yoga helps alleviate muscle imbalances and tension that contribute to poor posture by targeting areas of tightness and weakness in the body, releasing tension and promoting muscular relaxation. Chair yoga also encourages seniors to pay attention to their posture throughout the day, leading to conscious adjustments to their posture, both during yoga practice and in everyday activities.

Improved posture through chair yoga can have far-reaching benefits for overall health and well-being, including reduced risk of musculoskeletal issues such as back pain and neck strain, enhanced respiratory function, digestion, and circulation.

Additionally, studies suggest that upright posture can positively impact mood and self-confidence, leading to greater feelings of vitality and well-being.

Overall, chair yoga offers seniors a holistic approach to improving posture, addressing the interconnectedness of physical alignment, muscular strength, and body awareness.

7. Enhanced Mental Clarity:

Improving posture is crucial for the overall health and well-being of seniors, and chair yoga is of course an effective method for achieving this. Chair yoga poses are specifically designed to promote spinal alignment and enhance core strength, which are key factors in maintaining good posture.

With regular practice, seniors can notice significant improvements in their posture, with their shoulders back, chest open, and spine elongated. Chair yoga also strengthens the muscles that support good posture, especially the core muscles, which are essential for maintaining proper alignment and posture.

Furthermore, it targets areas of tightness and weakness in the body, releasing tension and promoting muscular relaxation, thus alleviating muscle imbalances and tension that contribute to poor posture. By encouraging seniors to pay attention to their posture throughout the day, chair yoga helps them make conscious adjustments to their posture, both during yoga practice and in everyday activities.

Improved posture through chair yoga can have numerous benefits for seniors, including a reduced risk of musculoskeletal issues such as back pain and neck strain, and improved respiratory function, digestion, and circulation. Studies suggest that upright posture can positively impact mood and self-confidence, leading to greater feelings of vitality and well-being. All in all, chair yoga offers seniors a holistic approach to improving posture, addressing the interconnectedness of physical alignment, muscular strength, and body awareness.

8. Social Connection:

Connecting with others is essential to our well-being, especially as we age. Chair yoga can offer seniors a unique opportunity to come together in an inclusive and supportive environment, fostering friendships and a sense of community.

By practicing yoga together, seniors can offer support, encouragement, and camaraderie, strengthening social bonds and promoting social connection. Chair yoga classes provide a safe and inclusive space for seniors of all abilities and backgrounds to come together, fostering a sense of acceptance and belonging, which can help reduce feelings of loneliness and isolation.

Also, chair yoga classes allow seniors to engage in meaningful activities and pursue shared interests beyond the yoga studio, inspiring them to come together and make a positive impact. Through shared laughter, encouragement, and mutual support, seniors can find strength, resilience, and comfort in each other's company, enriching their lives and enhancing their sense of connection.

Chapter 3:

Getting Started: Setting Up Your Space

1. Creating a Comfortable Environment
2. Gathering Essential Equipment
3. Setting the Mood
4. Preparing Mentally and Emotionally
5. Practising Safety Precautions
6. Establishing a Consistent Routine

1. Creating a Comfortable Environment:

- Select a room or area in your home that is free from distractions and noise.

- Aim for natural light if possible, or use soft lighting to create a calming ambiance.

- Arrange your furniture in a way that allows for easy movement and accessibility during practice.

- Ensure that your chair is positioned on a stable surface and that there is enough space around it for stretching and reaching comfortably.

- Choose a chair that is sturdy and provides adequate support for your body.

- Look for a chair with a straight back and armrests for added stability and comfort.

- Add elements that contribute to a sense of comfort and relaxation, such as cushions or blankets for added support and warmth.

- Consider incorporating personal items or decorations that bring you joy and create a welcoming atmosphere in your practice space.

- Turn off electronic devices or set them to silent mode to minimize distractions during your practice.

- Inform family members or housemates of your practice time and ask for their cooperation in maintaining a quiet environment.

2. Gathering Essential Equipment:

- Your yoga mat serves as your foundation, providing traction and stability during your practice. Opt for a high-quality mat or non-slip surface to prevent slips and ensure safety.

- Choose clothing that allows for ease of movement and breathability. Look for stretchy, moisture-wicking fabrics that won't restrict your mobility as you flow through poses.

- Hydration is key to a successful yoga practice. Keep a water bottle nearby to stay hydrated and replenish fluids throughout your session.

- Consider incorporating props such as bolsters, cushions, or blocks to support your practice and enhance comfort. These props can provide additional stability and assistance in achieving proper alignment in your poses.

3. Setting the Mood:

- Dim the lights or opt for soft, gentle lighting to create a calming atmosphere. Consider using candles or fairy lights to add a touch of warmth and tranquility to your space.

- Choose soothing music or nature sounds to accompany your practice and help you unwind. Look for instrumental tracks or nature sounds like ocean waves or birdsong that promote relaxation and mindfulness.

- Incorporate the power of scent to enhance your practice with aromatherapy. Use essential oils or scented candles with calming scents like lavender, chamomile, or eucalyptus to create a peaceful and inviting environment.

- Clear away any clutter or distractions from your practice area to create a sense of openness and serenity. A tidy space will help you focus your attention and fully immerse yourself in the present moment.

- Designate your practice area as a sacred space dedicated to self-care and mindfulness. Add meaningful decorations or symbols that inspire you and bring a sense of peace and intention to your practice.

4. Preparing Mentally and Emotionally:

- Take a few moments to reflect on what you hope to achieve during your practice. Whether it's finding peace, reducing stress, or improving flexibility, setting intentions can help focus your mind and guide your practice.

- Begin your practice with a grateful heart by acknowledging the blessings in your life. Expressing gratitude can shift your perspective and create a positive mindset that enhances your overall well-being.

- Release any expectations or judgments you may have about your practice. Allow yourself to be present in the moment and embrace whatever arises with openness and acceptance.

- Take a few deep breaths to center yourself and bring your awareness to the present moment. Pay attention to the rhythm of your breath as you inhale and exhale, allowing it to anchor you in the here and now.

- Be kind and gentle with yourself throughout your practice. Let go of perfectionism and embrace self-compassion as you navigate your yoga journey.

- Visualize yourself moving through your practice with ease and grace.

Envision yourself achieving your goals and feeling a sense of accomplishment and fulfillment.

5. Practicing Safety Precautions

- Pay attention to how your body feels during each pose and movement. If you experience any pain or discomfort, ease out of the pose or modify it to better suit your needs.

- Respect your body's limits and avoid pushing yourself too hard. Take breaks as needed and honor your body's signals to prevent strain or injury.

- Don't hesitate to modify poses to accommodate any physical limitations or injuries you may have. Use props or adjust the pose to make it more accessible and comfortable for your body.

- Begin your practice with gentle warm-up exercises to prepare your body for movement. Focus on gradually increasing flexibility and mobility in your joints and muscles.

- Drink water before, during, and after your practice to stay hydrated and replenish fluids lost through sweat. Dehydration can lead to fatigue and decreased performance, so make hydration a priority.

- Utilize props such as blocks, straps, or cushions to support your body and maintain proper alignment in poses. Props can help you safely deepen your practice and prevent injury.

- Practice in a clear, open space free from obstacles or hazards. Ensure that your chair is stable and placed on a non-slip surface to prevent falls or accidents.

- If you have any pre-existing medical conditions or concerns, consult with your healthcare provider before starting a new exercise routine. They can offer guidance and recommendations tailored to your individual needs.

6. Establishing a Consistent Routine

- Schedule regular time slots for your chair yoga practice, ideally at the same time each day or week. Treat these appointments with yourself as non-negotiable commitments to prioritize your well-being.

- Develop a pre-practice ritual to signal the start of your yoga session. This could include lighting a candle, practicing a few moments of deep breathing, or setting an intention for your practice.

- Begin with shorter practice sessions, such as 10-15 minutes, and gradually increase the duration as you build strength and endurance. Consistency is more important than intensity, so focus on showing up regularly, even if it's for a brief practice.

- Keep your practice fresh and engaging by incorporating variety into your routine. Explore different chair yoga sequences, styles, or instructors to prevent boredom and challenge yourself in new ways.

- Keep a journal or log of your chair yoga practice to track your progress over time. Note any changes in how you feel physically, mentally, or emotionally, as well as any milestones or achievements you reach along the way.

- Enlist the support of a friend, family member, or accountability partner to help you stay committed to your practice. Share your goals and progress with them, and check in regularly to celebrate successes and troubleshoot challenges together.

- Life can be unpredictable, so be prepared to adapt your practice schedule as needed. If you miss a session or encounter obstacles, don't be discouraged—simply adjust your plans and resume your practice when possible.

- Acknowledge and celebrate your dedication to establishing a consistent chair yoga routine. Recognize the positive impact it has on your health, happiness, and overall well-being, and take pride in your commitment to self-care.

By adhering to these space-setting recommendations, you'll create an inviting and supportive environment for your chair yoga practice, laying the groundwork for a rewarding and engaging path toward better health and wellness.

Chapter 4: Exploring Chair Yoga Poses

1. Seated Mountain Pose

- Sit comfortably in your chair with your feet flat on the floor and your spine tall and elongated. Ground down through your sit bones, feeling a sense of stability and support from the earth beneath you.

- Draw your navel gently in towards your spine to activate your core muscles. This engagement helps to stabilize your pelvis and spine, promoting proper alignment and posture.

- Imagine a string pulling you up from the crown of your head towards the sky, lengthening your spine and creating space between each vertebra. Feel a sense of openness and expansiveness in your chest and shoulders.

- Soften your shoulders away from your ears, allowing them to melt down and back. Feel tension releasing from your neck and shoulders as you find a sense of ease and relaxation.

- Soften your gaze and fix your eyes on a point in front of you, maintaining a steady focus and presence. This helps to calm the mind and cultivate a sense of inner stillness and concentration.

- Take slow, deep breaths, filling your lungs with air and exhaling fully. Allow your breath to flow naturally and effortlessly, anchoring you in the present moment and connecting you to the rhythm of life.

- Finally, simply be. Allow yourself to surrender to the moment, letting go of the need to do or achieve anything. Find peace in the stillness, knowing that you are grounded, stable, and strong, just like the mountain.

2. Seated Forward Bend: Embracing Relaxation and Surrender

- Sit comfortably in your chair with your feet flat on the floor and your spine tall and elongated. Ground down through your sit bones, feeling rooted and supported.

- On an inhale, elongate your spine, lifting your chest towards the sky. Feel a gentle stretch along your spine as you create space between each vertebra.

- On an exhale, begin to fold forward from your hips, leading with your heart. Keep your spine long as you fold, avoiding rounding your back.

- Allow your arms to dangle towards the floor or reach for your feet or shins, depending on your flexibility. Let go of any tension in your neck, shoulders, and jaw as you surrender into the pose.

- Take slow, deep breaths, allowing your breath to guide you deeper into the pose with each exhale. Feel the gentle stretch in your hamstrings and lower back with each breath.

- Soften your gaze and bring your awareness to the sensations in your body. Notice any areas of tightness or resistance, and gently breathe into them, allowing them to release and soften.

- Allow yourself to surrender fully into the pose, letting go of any thoughts or distractions. Find peace in the stillness and embrace the sense of relaxation and calm that washes over you.

- Remain in the pose for several breaths, enjoying the deep stretch and relaxation it provides. When you're ready to release, slowly rise back up to a seated position with a tall spine.

3. Seated Twist

- Begin by sitting comfortably in your chair with your feet flat on the floor and your spine tall and elongated.

Ground down through your sit bones, feeling stable and rooted.

- On an inhale, lift your arms overhead, reaching towards the sky. Feel a gentle stretch along the sides of your body as you lengthen your spine.

- On an exhale, bring your right hand to the outside of your left knee, gently twisting your torso to the right. Place your left hand on the back of the chair for support and stability.

- Engage your core muscles to support your spine as you deepen the twist. Imagine wringing out any tension or toxins from your internal organs with each breath.

- Take slow, deep breaths as you hold the twist, allowing your breath to guide you deeper into the pose with each exhale. Feel the gentle twist along your spine and the opening in your chest.

- Soften your gaze and bring your awareness to the sensations in your body. Notice the stretch in your back, shoulders, and hips, and breathe into any areas of tightness or resistance.

- After several breaths, gently release the twist and return to center. Take a moment to pause and observe the effects of the pose before repeating the twist on the opposite side.

4. Seated Cat-Cow Stretch

- Begin by sitting comfortably in your chair with your feet flat on the floor and your spine tall and elongated. Place your hands on your knees or thighs for support.

- On an inhale, gently arch your spine, lifting your chest and heart towards the sky. Allow your belly to sink towards the floor as you broaden across your collarbones.

- On an exhale, round your spine like a Halloween cat, drawing your belly button towards your spine and tucking your chin towards your chest. Feel the stretch along your back as you press firmly into your hands and feet.

- Continue to flow between Cow Pose and Cat Pose with each inhale and exhale, moving with the rhythm of your breath. Allow the movement to be fluid and intuitive, syncing your breath with your body's natural rhythm.

- As you flow through the sequence, explore variations such as circling your torso in one direction and then the other, or adding gentle side bends to further open up your side body.

- Soften your gaze and bring your awareness to the sensations in your body as you move through the sequence. Notice the subtle shifts in your spine and the connection between your breath and movement.

- After several rounds, return to a neutral spine and take a moment to rest and observe the effects of the Cat-Cow Stretch. Notice any changes in your breath, posture, or overall sense of well-being.

5. Seated Side Stretch

- Begin by sitting comfortably in your chair with your feet flat on the floor and your spine tall and elongated. Root down through your sit bones and engage your core for stability.

- On an inhale, reach both arms overhead, lengthening through your fingertips towards the sky. Feel a gentle stretch along the sides of your body as you create space between each rib.

- On an exhale, lower your right arm down towards the floor, keeping your left arm extended overhead. Keep both sit bones grounded as you stretch through the left side of your body.

- Engage your abdominal muscles to support your spine and deepen the stretch. Imagine drawing your navel towards your spine to maintain stability and alignment.

- Take slow, deep breaths as you hold the stretch, allowing your breath to guide you deeper into the pose with each exhale. Feel the expansion in your ribcage and the opening in your heart.

- Soften your gaze and bring your awareness to the sensations in your body. Notice the stretch along the left side of your body and any areas of tightness or resistance.

- Remain in the stretch for several breaths, enjoying the lengthening and opening it provides. When you're ready to release, inhale to return to center and exhale to repeat the stretch on the opposite side.

Chapter 5

Breathing Techniques for Relaxation

1. Deep Belly Breathing (Diaphragmatic Breathing):

- Sit comfortably in your chair with your feet flat on the floor and your hands resting on your abdomen. Inhale deeply through your nose, allowing your belly to expand fully. Exhale slowly through your mouth, drawing your navel towards your spine. Repeat for several breaths, focusing on the sensation of your breath filling your belly and chest.

2. 4-7-8 Breathing (Relaxation Breath):

- Begin by exhaling completely through your mouth, making a whooshing sound. Close your mouth and inhale quietly through your nose for a count of four. Hold your breath for a count of seven. Exhale slowly through your mouth for a count of eight, making a whooshing sound. Repeat this cycle for four rounds, allowing each breath to deepen your relaxation.

3. Equal Breathing (Sama Vritti):

- Inhale slowly and steadily through your nose for a count of four. Exhale through your nose for a count of four, matching the length of your inhale. Repeat this pattern for several rounds, focusing on creating a smooth and even rhythm with your breath. As you continue, you may gradually increase the length of your inhales and exhales if comfortable.

4. Alternate Nostril Breathing (Nadi Shodhana):

- Sit comfortably with your spine tall and your left hand resting on your left knee. Bring your right hand to your face and place your index and middle fingers between your eyebrows.

Close your right nostril with your right thumb and inhale deeply through your left nostril. Close your left nostril with your ring finger and exhale fully through your right nostril. Inhale through your right nostril, then close it with your thumb and exhale through your left nostril. Continue this pattern for several rounds, alternating nostrils with each breath.

Chapter 6:

Chair Yoga Sequences for Flexibility

Morning Routine: Energize and Invigorate Your Day

1. Seated Cat-Cow Stretch:

- Begin by sitting comfortably in your chair with your feet flat on the floor and your hands resting on your knees. Inhale as you arch your back (Cow Pose), lifting your chest and heart towards the sky. Exhale as you round your spine (Cat Pose), tucking your chin towards your chest. Repeat this flowing movement for several rounds, synchronizing your breath with your movement to gently awaken your spine and increase flexibility.

2. Seated Forward Fold:

- Inhale as you lengthen your spine, reaching your arms overhead. Exhale as you hinge forward from your hips, folding your torso towards your thighs. Allow your hands to rest on your shins or the floor, and let your head hang heavy. Take several deep breaths in this position, feeling the stretch along the back of your body and the release of tension in your spine and hamstrings.

3. Seated Side Stretch:

- Inhale as you reach your arms overhead, lengthening through your fingertips. Exhale as you lean to the right, stretching the left side of your body. Hold for a few breaths, feeling the gentle opening along your side. Inhale to return to center, then exhale to repeat the stretch on the opposite side. Continue to flow between each side, breathing deeply and finding a sense of spaciousness in your body.

4. Seated Twist:

- Inhale to lengthen your spine, then exhale to twist towards the right, placing your left hand on your right knee and your right hand on the back of your chair. Hold the twist for a few breaths, feeling the gentle rotation in your spine and the detoxifying effect on your organs. Inhale to return to center, then exhale to repeat the twist on the left side. Continue to alternate between each side, breathing deeply and allowing each twist to wring out tension and promote flexibility.

5. Deep Breathing:

- Close your eyes and take several deep breaths, inhaling through your nose and exhaling through your mouth. Allow each breath to fill you with a sense of vitality and renewal, energizing your body and calming your mind. Take a moment to express gratitude for the day ahead and set positive intentions for the hours to come.

Afternoon Stretch: Renew and Revitalize Your Body

1. Seated Shoulder Rolls:

- Sit comfortably in your chair with your feet flat on the floor and your hands resting on your thighs. Inhale as you lift your shoulders towards your ears, then exhale as you roll them back and down. Repeat this movement several times, allowing each roll to release tension and create space in your shoulders.

2. Seated Side Bend:

- Inhale as you reach your right arm overhead, stretching towards the left side. Keep your left hand grounded on the chair for support and avoid collapsing into the stretch. Hold for a few breaths, feeling the gentle opening along the right side of your body. Exhale to release and switch sides. Repeat on each side to release tension and increase flexibility in your side body.

3. Seated Forward Fold with Chest Expansion:

- Inhale as you lengthen your spine, then exhale as you hinge forward from your hips, folding your torso towards your thighs. Interlace your fingers behind your back and gently straighten your arms as you lift them towards the sky, opening your chest and shoulders. Hold for a few breaths, feeling the stretch in your hamstrings, spine, and chest. Exhale to release and slowly return to an upright position.

4. Seated Spinal Twist:

- Inhale to lengthen your spine, then exhale to twist towards the right, placing your left hand on the outside of your right knee and your right hand on the back of your chair. Hold the twist for a few breaths, feeling the gentle rotation in your spine and the release of tension in your back. Inhale to return to center, then exhale to twist to the left. Repeat on each side to relieve stiffness and improve spinal mobility.

5. Deep Breathing and Mindful Rest:

- Close your eyes and take several deep breaths, inhaling deeply through your nose and exhaling fully through your mouth. Allow each breath to bring a sense of relaxation and calm to your body and mind. Take a moment to appreciate yourself for taking this time to care for your well-being and recharge your energy.

Evening Relaxation: Unwind and Restore Your Body

1. Seated Neck Stretch:

- Sit comfortably in your chair with your spine tall and your shoulders relaxed. Gently tilt your head to the right, bringing your right ear towards your right shoulder. Place your right hand on the left side of your head and apply gentle pressure to deepen the stretch. Hold for a few breaths, then switch sides. Repeat on each side to release tension in your neck and shoulders.

2. Seated Heart Opener:

- Inhale as you reach your arms behind you, interlacing your fingers and opening your chest towards the sky. Lift your gaze slightly and draw your shoulder blades together to deepen the stretch in your chest and shoulders. Hold for a few breaths, feeling the gentle expansion across your heart center. Exhale to release and return to a neutral position.

3. Seated Forward Fold with Gentle Twist:

- Inhale to lengthen your spine, then exhale as you hinge forward from your hips, folding your torso towards your thighs. Allow your arms to hang loosely or rest them on your legs for support. Take a few breaths in this forward fold, feeling the release of tension in your spine and hamstrings.

On your next exhale, twist gently to the right, placing your left hand on your right knee and your right hand on the back of your chair. Hold for a few breaths, then return to center and repeat on the left side. Alternate between forward fold and gentle twist, allowing each movement to deepen your relaxation.

4. Seated Pigeon Pose:

- Sit towards the edge of your chair and cross your right ankle over your left knee, flexing your right foot to protect your knee. Keep your spine tall as you gently lean forward, feeling the stretch in your right hip and glute. Hold for a few breaths, then switch sides. Repeat on each side to release tension and increase flexibility in your hips and lower back.

5. Deep Breathing and Mindful Release:

- Close your eyes and take several deep breaths, inhaling deeply through your nose and exhaling fully through your mouth. Allow each breath to bring a sense of calm and relaxation to your body and mind. Release any tension or stress with each exhale, allowing yourself to fully let go and surrender to the present moment.

Chapter 7

Leg Strengthening Exercises: Build Stability and Power

1. Chair Pose (Utkatasana Variation):

- Begin by sitting towards the edge of your chair with your feet hip-width apart and your knees aligned over your ankles. Inhale as you reach your arms overhead, palms facing each other. Exhale as you bend your knees and lower your hips towards the ground, as if sitting back into an imaginary chair. Hold for several breaths, engaging your quadriceps and glutes to support your lower body. Inhale to rise back up to a standing position, then repeat for several rounds to strengthen your legs and build endurance.

2. Standing Knee Lifts:

- Stand behind your chair with your feet hip-width apart and your hands resting lightly on the backrest for support. Inhale as you lift your right knee towards your chest, engaging your core and quadriceps. Hold for a few breaths, then exhale to lower your foot back down. Repeat on the left side, alternating between each leg for several rounds. Focus on lifting with control and maintaining stability through your standing leg to strengthen your thighs and improve balance.

3. Warrior II (Virabhadrasana II Variation):

- Sit towards the edge of your chair with your feet wide apart and your right knee bent at a 90-degree angle, aligning with your ankle. Extend your left leg behind you, keeping it straight and engaged. Inhale as you reach your arms out to the sides, parallel to the floor, with your palms facing down.

  Exhale as you gaze over your right fingertips, sinking deeper into your right knee. Hold for several breaths, feeling the strength and stability in your legs and the stretch in your inner thighs and hips. Inhale to rise back up, then switch sides and repeat on the left.

4. Leg Extensions:

- Sit tall in your chair with your feet flat on the floor and your hands resting on your thighs. Inhale as you extend your right leg straight out in front of you, engaging your quadriceps and pressing through your heel. Hold for a few breaths, then exhale to lower your foot back down. Repeat on the left side, alternating between each leg for several rounds. Focus on maintaining good posture and control throughout the movement to strengthen your thighs and improve knee stability.

5. Bridge Pose (Setu Bandhasana Variation):

- Sit towards the edge of your chair with your feet hip-width apart and your knees bent at a 90-degree angle. Place your hands on the sides of your chair for support. Inhale as you press down through your feet and lift your hips towards the sky, creating a straight line from your knees to your shoulders. Engage your glutes and thighs as you hold the pose for several breaths, feeling the strength and stability in your lower body. Exhale to lower your hips back down to the chair. Repeat for several rounds to build strength and endurance in your legs and hips.

Arm Strengthening Exercises: Build Upper Body Strength

1. Chair Dips:

- Begin by sitting on the edge of your chair with your hands gripping the front edge, fingers pointing forward. Walk your feet forward until your hips are just in front of the chair. Inhale to bend your elbows, lowering your hips towards the floor. Exhale to press through your palms, straightening your arms and lifting your hips back up. Repeat for several rounds, focusing on engaging your triceps and keeping your core stable to strengthen your arms and shoulders.

2. Seated Shoulder Press:

-   Sit tall in your chair with your feet flat on the floor and your spine elongated. Hold a lightweight object, such as a water bottle or small dumbbell, in each hand at shoulder height, palms facing forward. Inhale as you press the weights overhead, extending your arms fully without locking your elbows. Exhale as you lower the weights back down to shoulder height. Repeat for several rounds, focusing on controlled movements and engaging your shoulder muscles to build strength and stability.

3. Chair Plank Hold:

-   Begin by sitting towards the edge of your chair with your hands gripping the front edge, fingers pointing forward. Walk your feet back until your body forms a straight line from your head to your heels, with your arms supporting your weight. Engage your core and squeeze your glutes to maintain stability. Hold this plank position for several breaths, focusing on keeping your body aligned and your muscles engaged to strengthen your arms, shoulders, and core.

4. Chair Tricep Extensions:

- Sit tall in your chair with your feet flat on the floor and your spine elongated. Hold a lightweight object, such as a water bottle or small dumbbell, in your right hand, extending it overhead. Inhale as you bend your right elbow, lowering the weight behind your head. Exhale as you straighten your arm, pressing the weight back up towards the ceiling.

Repeat for several rounds on the right side, then switch to the left. Focus on keeping your elbow stable and your movements controlled to effectively target and strengthen your triceps.

5. Seated Bicep Curls:

- Sit tall in your chair with your feet flat on the floor and your spine elongated. Hold a lightweight object, such as a water bottle or small dumbbell, in each hand, palms facing forward. Inhale as you bend your elbows, curling the weights towards your shoulders. Exhale as you lower the weights back down to your sides. Repeat for several rounds, focusing on squeezing your biceps at the top of the movement and maintaining good posture to effectively strengthen your arms.

Core Stability Poses: Strengthen Your Center

1. Seated Spinal Twist:

- Sit tall in your chair with your feet flat on the floor and your spine elongated. Inhale as you lengthen your spine, then exhale as you twist towards the right, placing your left hand on the outside of your right knee and your right hand on the back of your chair. Use your breath to deepen the twist, engaging your core muscles to support your spine. Hold for several breaths, then inhale to return to center and exhale to repeat on the left side. Alternate between each side to strengthen and mobilize your spine while engaging your core.

2. Chair Boat Pose:

- Sit towards the edge of your chair with your knees bent and your feet flat on the floor. Hold onto the sides of your chair for support as you lean back slightly, lifting your feet off the ground. Engage your core muscles to maintain balance and stability as you straighten your legs and extend them forward, creating a V shape with your body. Hold for several breaths, feeling the engagement in your abdominals and hip flexors. Exhale to lower your feet back down to the floor. Repeat for several rounds to strengthen your core and improve balance.

3. Seated Cat-Cow Stretch with Core Engagement:

- Begin in a seated position with your feet flat on the floor and your hands resting on your thighs. Inhale as you arch your back and lift your chest towards the sky (Cow Pose), engaging your core muscles to support your spine. Exhale as you round your spine and tuck your chin towards your chest (Cat Pose), drawing your navel towards your spine. Continue to flow between Cat and Cow poses, linking your breath with your movement and focusing on engaging your core throughout the entire sequence to strengthen and stabilize your abdominal muscles.

4. Chair Plank Pose:

- Sit towards the edge of your chair with your hands gripping the front edge, fingers pointing forward. Walk your feet back until your body forms a straight line from your head to your heels, with your arms supporting your weight. Engage your core muscles and hold this plank position for several breaths, focusing on maintaining a strong and stable alignment from head to heels. Keep your shoulders stacked over your wrists and avoid sinking into your lower back. Exhale to release and return to a seated position. Repeat for several rounds to build strength and stability in your core muscles.

5. Seated Leg Lifts:

- Sit tall in your chair with your feet flat on the floor and your hands resting on your thighs. Inhale as you lift your right leg off the floor, extending it straight out in front of you while engaging your core muscles to maintain stability. Hold for several breaths, then exhale to lower your foot back down. Repeat on the left side, alternating between each leg for several rounds. Focus on keeping your spine tall and your core engaged throughout the movement to strengthen your abdominals and improve stability.

Chapter 8

Chair yoga for Joints

1. Chair Hip Flexion and Extension:

- Sit tall in a sturdy chair with your feet flat on the floor and knees bent at a 90-degree angle.

- Begin by lifting your right knee towards your chest, flexing your hip. Hold for a moment, then extend your right leg forward, straightening your knee.

- Repeat this movement, alternating between hip flexion and extension on each leg. Aim for 8-10 repetitions on each side.

2. Seated Knee Lifts:

- Sit upright in your chair with your feet flat on the floor.

- Slowly lift your right knee towards your chest, keeping your foot flexed and your back straight.

- Hold the lifted position for a few seconds, then gently lower your foot back to the floor.
- Repeat on the left side, alternating between each leg for 8-10 repetitions.

3. Chair Knee Extensions:

- Sit tall in your chair with your feet flat on the floor and knees bent at a 90-degree angle.

- Extend your right leg forward, straightening your knee as much as possible without locking it.

- Hold the extended position for a few seconds, then slowly lower your foot back to the floor.

- Repeat with your left leg, alternating between each leg for 8-10 repetitions.

4. Chair Hip Circles:

- Sit comfortably in your chair with your feet flat on the floor and hands resting on your thighs.

- Begin by circling your hips in a clockwise direction, making smooth and controlled movements.

- After several circles, reverse the direction and circle your hips counterclockwise.

- Continue alternating between clockwise and counterclockwise hip circles for 8-10 repetitions each.

5. Chair Knee Raises with Resistance Band:

- Sit tall in your chair with a resistance band looped around both thighs, just above your knees.

- Keep your feet flat on the floor and knees bent at a 90-degree angle.

- Engage your core and slowly lift your right knee towards your chest, pressing against the resistance band.

- Hold for a moment, then lower your foot back to the floor.

- Repeat with your left knee, alternating between each leg for 8-10 repetitions.

6. Gentle Shoulder Rolls:

- Sit comfortably in your chair with your feet flat on the floor and hands resting on your thighs.

- Inhale as you lift your shoulders up towards your ears, then exhale as you roll them back and down in a smooth, circular motion.

- Repeat this movement for several rounds, focusing on releasing tension and promoting mobility in the shoulder joints.

7. Wrist Circles with Gentle Resistance:

- Sit comfortably in your chair with your feet flat on the floor and hands resting on your thighs.

- Extend your arms forward at shoulder height, palms facing down.

- Begin to make gentle circles with your wrists, moving in a clockwise direction while applying gentle resistance with your opposite hand.

- After several circles, reverse the direction and circle your wrists counterclockwise while maintaining gentle resistance.

- Continue alternating between clockwise and counterclockwise wrist circles with resistance for 8-10 repetitions each.

8. Ankle Rolls with Ankle Circles:

- Sit upright in your chair with your feet flat on the floor.

- Start by rolling your ankles in a circular motion, moving clockwise several times.

- Then, reverse the direction and roll your ankles counterclockwise for several repetitions.

- Next, extend your right leg forward and draw circles with your toes, moving clockwise several times.

- Reverse the direction and draw circles counterclockwise with your toes.

- Repeat the ankle circles with your left foot, alternating between clockwise and counterclockwise rotations.

Neck & Shoulder Relief

1. Neck Rolls:

- Sit comfortably in your chair with your feet flat on the floor and hands resting on your thighs.

- Inhale deeply and as you exhale, gently drop your chin towards your chest.

- Slowly roll your head to the right, bringing your right ear towards your right shoulder.

- Continue rolling your head back, bringing your chin towards the ceiling, then to the left, and finally back to the starting position.

- Repeat this movement in a smooth, circular motion for several rounds, then switch directions.

2. Shoulder Shrugs:

- Sit tall in your chair with your feet flat on the floor and arms relaxed by your sides.

- Inhale deeply and as you exhale, shrug your shoulders up towards your ears.

- Hold the shrug for a moment, then slowly release your shoulders back down.

- Repeat this movement for several repetitions, focusing on releasing tension in the shoulders with each exhale.

3. Shoulder Rolls:

- Sit comfortably in your chair with your feet flat on the floor and hands resting on your thighs.

- Inhale deeply and as you exhale, roll your shoulders back in a smooth, circular motion.

- Continue rolling your shoulders back for several repetitions, then switch directions and roll them forward.

- Focus on releasing tension and promoting mobility in the shoulder joints with each roll.

4. Neck Stretch:

- Sit tall in your chair with your feet flat on the floor and hands resting on your thighs.

- Reach your right hand towards the left side of your head and gently guide your right ear towards your right shoulder.

- Hold the stretch for a few deep breaths, feeling the gentle stretch along the side of your neck and shoulder.

- Repeat the stretch on the opposite side, reaching your left hand towards the right side of your head.

- Hold for a few breaths, then release and return to the starting position.

5. Eagle Arms Stretch:

- Sit tall in your chair with your feet flat on the floor and arms relaxed by your sides.

- Inhale as you extend your arms out to the sides at shoulder height.

- Exhale as you cross your right arm over your left, bending both elbows and bringing your palms together if possible.

- Hold the stretch for a few deep breaths, feeling the opening in the upper back and shoulders.

- Repeat the stretch on the opposite side, crossing your left arm over your right.

Chapter 9

Mindfulness and Meditation Practices

Guided Breathing Technique

1. Deep Breathing Exercise:

- Sit comfortably in your chair with your feet flat on the floor and hands resting on your thighs.

- Close your eyes and take a few deep breaths, inhaling through your nose and exhaling through your mouth.

- As you breathe, focus on the sensation of the breath entering and leaving your body, allowing each inhale to fill you with a sense of calm and each exhale to release any tension or stress.

2. Progressive Muscle Relaxation:

- Starting with your feet, tense the muscles in your toes and feet as tightly as you can for a few seconds.

- Then, slowly release the tension and let your muscles relax completely.

- Move up to your calves, thighs, abdomen, chest, arms, and finally your face, tensing and then relaxing each muscle group in turn.

- As you release the tension from each muscle group, imagine any stress or tension melting away, leaving you feeling deeply relaxed and at ease.

3. Body Scan Meditation:

- Close your eyes and take a few deep breaths to center yourself.

- Begin to bring your awareness to different parts of your body, starting with your toes and slowly moving up through your feet, ankles, legs, and so on, all the way up to the top of your head.

- As you focus on each part of your body, notice any sensations you may be experiencing, whether it's tension, discomfort, or relaxation.

- With each breath, imagine sending a wave of relaxation to that part of your body, allowing any tension or discomfort to dissolve away.

4. Guided Imagery:

- Close your eyes and take a few deep breaths to relax your body and mind.

- Picture yourself in a peaceful and serene setting, such as a beautiful beach, a tranquil forest, or a cozy mountain cabin.

- Use all of your senses to imagine the sights, sounds, smells, and sensations of this place, allowing yourself to fully immerse in the experience.

- As you continue to visualize this peaceful scene, feel your body becoming more and more relaxed, letting go of any stress or tension you may be holding onto.

5. Affirmations and Mantras:

- Choose a positive affirmation or mantra that resonates with you, such as "I am calm and at peace" or "I am relaxed and present in this moment."

- Close your eyes and repeat the affirmation or mantra to yourself silently or out loud, allowing the words to sink in and fill you with a sense of calm and relaxation.

- Continue to repeat the affirmation or mantra for a few minutes, focusing on the positive feelings it evokes within you.

Mindful Breathing Meditation

- Sit comfortably in your chair with your feet flat on the floor and hands resting on your thighs. Close your eyes or soften your gaze.

- Begin by bringing your awareness to your breath. Notice the natural rhythm of your breath as it flows in and out of your body.

- Take a slow, deep breath in through your nose, allowing your belly to expand as you fill your lungs with air. Count to four as you inhale.

- At the top of your inhale, gently hold your breath for a moment. Count to two at the top of your breath, savoring the fullness of the breath.

- Slowly exhale through your mouth, allowing your belly to gently contract as you release the air from your lungs. Count to four as you exhale.

- Continue this cycle of deep belly breathing, inhaling deeply through your nose, holding your breath briefly, and exhaling slowly through your mouth.

- As you breathe, keep your attention focused on the sensation of the breath moving in and out of your body. Notice the rise and fall of your belly with each inhale and exhale.

- With each exhale, imagine releasing any tension or stress you may be holding in your body. Allow yourself to relax more deeply with each breath.

- If your mind starts to wander, gently bring your attention back to your breath. Let go of any thoughts or distractions, and simply be present with the sensation of breathing.

- Practice this mindful breathing meditation for several minutes, allowing yourself to sink deeper into a state of relaxation with each breath.

- When you're ready to end the meditation, take a few more deep breaths, and gently open your eyes. Take a moment to acknowledge yourself for taking this time for self-care and gratitude for your breath and well-being.

Visualization Exercises

- Find a comfortable seated position in your chair, ensuring that your feet are flat on the floor and your spine is comfortably upright. Close your eyes or soften your gaze.

- Begin by taking a few deep breaths to relax your body and calm your mind. Inhale deeply through your nose, filling your lungs with air, and exhale slowly through your mouth, releasing any tension or stress.

- Visualize yourself in a peaceful and serene setting of your choice. It could be a beautiful beach, a tranquil forest, a peaceful garden, or any other place where you feel safe and at ease.

- Use all of your senses to fully immerse yourself in this imagined scene. Notice the colors, shapes, and textures around you. Listen to the sounds of nature, whether it's the gentle rustling of leaves, the soothing sound of ocean waves, or the chirping of birds.

- Begin to explore your surroundings in your mind's eye. Walk along a path, feel the warmth of the sun on your skin, and breathe in the fresh, clean air. Notice any sensations of peace, tranquility, and relaxation that arise within you.

- As you continue to visualize this peaceful scene, notice how it makes you feel. Allow yourself to fully experience feelings of calmness, serenity, and contentment washing over you.

- Whenever your mind starts to wander or thoughts arise, gently bring your focus back to the present moment and the visualization exercise. Let go of any distractions and fully immerse yourself in the experience.

- Spend a few moments simply savoring the experience of being in this peaceful place, allowing yourself to feel fully present and at peace.

- When you're ready to conclude the visualization exercise, take a few more deep breaths and gradually bring your awareness back to your physical surroundings.

- Slowly open your eyes and take a moment to reflect on the experience, feeling refreshed and rejuvenated.

Chapter 10

Chair Yoga For Better Sleep

1. Seated Spinal Twist:

- Sit tall in your chair with your feet flat on the floor.

- Inhale to lengthen your spine, then exhale as you twist your torso to the right, placing your left hand on the outside of your right knee and your right hand on the back of the chair.

- Hold the twist for a few breaths, feeling the gentle stretch along your spine.

- Inhale to return to center, then exhale as you twist to the left, repeating the stretch on the other side.

2. Gentle Shoulder Rolls:

- Sit comfortably in your chair with your feet flat on the floor and hands resting on your thighs.

- Inhale deeply and as you exhale, roll your shoulders back in a smooth, circular motion.

- Continue rolling your shoulders back for several repetitions, then switch directions and roll them forward.

- Focus on releasing tension and promoting relaxation in your shoulders and upper back.

3. Deep Breathing Exercise:

- Close your eyes and take a few deep breaths to center yourself.

- Inhale deeply through your nose, counting to four as you fill your lungs with air.

- Hold your breath for a moment, then exhale slowly through your mouth, counting to four as you release the air from your lungs.

- Continue this deep breathing pattern for several cycles, allowing each breath to relax you more deeply.

4. Seated Forward Bend:

- Sit tall in your chair with your feet flat on the floor and hands resting on your thighs.

- Inhale to lengthen your spine, then exhale as you hinge forward from your hips, bringing your chest towards your thighs.

- Allow your arms to hang loosely or reach towards the floor, depending on your flexibility.

- Hold the forward bend for a few deep breaths, feeling the stretch along your spine and the backs of your legs.

5. Guided Relaxation Meditation:

- Close your eyes and take a few deep breaths to relax your body and calm your mind.

- Visualize yourself in a peaceful and serene setting, such as a tranquil beach or a quiet forest.

- Use all of your senses to fully immerse yourself in this scene, noticing the sights, sounds, smells, and sensations around you.

- Spend a few minutes simply being present in this peaceful place, allowing yourself to relax and unwind fully.

6. Gratitude Practice:

- Take a moment to reflect on three things you're grateful for today. They can be simple things like a warm cup of tea or a phone call with a loved one.

- As you think about each thing you're grateful for, take a deep breath in and exhale slowly, feeling a sense of appreciation and contentment wash over you.

7. Closing Affirmation:

- End your wind-down routine with a positive affirmation or intention for the evening. It could be something like ***"I am grateful for the peace and relaxation I feel in this moment"*** or ***"I am ready to embrace a restful and rejuvenating night's sleep."***

Chapter 11

Chair Yoga Modifications and Props

Using Bolster And Cushions

1. Seated Meditation with Bolster Support:

- Place a bolster or cushion on the seat of the chair to provide extra padding and support.

- Sit comfortably on the bolster with your spine tall and shoulders relaxed.

- Allow your hands to rest on your thighs or in your lap, palms facing up or down.

- Close your eyes and focus on your breath, allowing the bolster to provide a stable and comfortable base for your meditation practice.

2. Supported Seated Forward Bend with Bolster:

- Sit towards the front of the chair with your feet flat on the floor and knees bent.

- Place a bolster or cushion on your lap, extending it forward over your legs.

- Inhale to lengthen your spine, then exhale as you hinge forward from your hips, allowing your torso to rest on the bolster.

- Support your head with your hands or allow it to rest on the bolster if comfortable.

- Hold the forward bend for a few deep breaths, feeling the gentle stretch along your spine and the release of tension in your lower back.

3. Supported Seated Twist with Bolster:

- Sit tall in your chair with your feet flat on the floor and knees bent.

- Place a bolster or cushion on the seat of the chair behind you.

- Inhale to lengthen your spine, then exhale as you twist your torso to the right, placing your left hand on the outside of your right knee and your right hand on the bolster behind you.

- Hold the twist for a few breaths, feeling the support of the bolster as you deepen the stretch in your spine and torso.

- Inhale to return to center, then exhale as you twist to the left, repeating the stretch on the other side.

4. Restorative Chest Opener with Cushions:

- Sit comfortably in your chair with your feet flat on the floor and hands resting on your thighs.

- Place one or more cushions vertically behind your back, allowing them to support your upper back and shoulders.

- Lean back against the cushions, allowing your chest to open and your shoulders to relax.

- You can keep your arms resting on your thighs or extend them out to the sides for a deeper stretch in your chest and shoulders.

- Close your eyes and take several deep breaths, allowing the cushions to provide gentle support as you open your heart and release tension in your upper body.

5. Supported Savasana with Bolster:

- Sit towards the front of the chair with your feet flat on the floor and knees bent.

- Place a bolster or cushion horizontally on the seat of the chair behind you.

- Lie back on the bolster, allowing it to support your spine from your lower back to your head.

- Extend your legs out in front of you or keep them bent with your feet flat on the floor, whichever is more comfortable.

- Close your eyes and relax completely, allowing the bolster to provide support and comfort as you surrender into the pose.

Adapting Poses For Mobility Challenges

1. **Seated Mountain Pose (Tadasana Variation):**

- For individuals with limited mobility in their arms or shoulders, keep the arms relaxed by their sides or resting on their thighs instead of reaching them overhead.

2. **Seated Forward Bend (Paschimottanasana Variation):**

- If reaching towards the floor is challenging, individuals can place their hands on their shins or knees, or simply let their arms hang down towards the floor for a gentle stretch.

3. Seated Twist:

- For those with limited spinal mobility, encourage gentle twists within their comfortable range of motion. They can also use the armrests of the chair for support while twisting.

4. Seated Cat-Cow Stretch:

- Individuals can focus on the pelvic tilts involved in the movement rather than rounding and arching their entire spine. They can also perform smaller, gentler movements if a full range of motion is not accessible.

5. Seated Side Stretch:

- Instead of reaching the arm overhead towards the opposite side, individuals can simply lean gently to one side while keeping the opposite arm relaxed by their side or resting on the chair.

6. Chair Pigeon Pose:

- For individuals with limited hip mobility, they can perform a modified version by crossing one ankle over the opposite knee and gently pressing down on the crossed knee to stretch the outer hip.

7. Chair Warrior Pose:

- Simplify the pose by keeping the feet hip-width apart and the knees bent at a comfortable angle. Instead of lifting the arms overhead, individuals can keep them by their sides or place them on their hips for stability.

8. Seated Tree Pose:

- Modify the pose by placing the foot on the inside of the calf or ankle instead of pressing it against the thigh. Individuals can also use the wall or chair for support if balancing is challenging.

9. Seated Eagle Pose:

- Simplify the pose by crossing one leg over the other at the ankles rather than wrapping the foot behind the calf. Individuals can focus on gently squeezing the legs together to engage the muscles.

10. Seated Savasana (Corpse Pose):

- Lie back comfortably in the chair with the feet flat on the floor and arms resting by the sides. Support the head and neck with a cushion or folded towel if needed for additional comfort.

Seated Yoga Strap Stretches

1. Seated Forward Fold with Strap:

- Sit comfortably on the edge of a chair with your legs extended in front of you and feet hip-width apart.

- Loop a yoga strap around the bottoms of your feet and hold one end of the strap in each hand.

- Inhale to lengthen your spine, then exhale as you hinge forward from your hips, keeping your back flat.

- Hold onto the strap as you fold forward, allowing your chest to come towards your thighs and your forehead to move towards your shins.

- Hold the stretch for several breaths, feeling the gentle opening in the backs of your legs and spine.

2. Seated Shoulder Stretch with Strap:

- Sit tall in your chair with your feet flat on the floor and knees hip-width apart.

- Hold the strap with both hands, keeping your arms extended in front of you at shoulder height.

- Inhale to lengthen your spine, then exhale as you slowly lift the strap overhead, keeping your arms straight.

- Once the strap is overhead, exhale and gently lower it behind your head, allowing your arms to bend slightly if needed.

- Hold the stretch for several breaths, feeling the opening across your chest and shoulders.

3. Seated Side Stretch with Strap:

- Sit comfortably on the edge of your chair with your feet flat on the floor and spine tall.

- Hold the strap with both hands, extending your arms overhead.

- Inhale to lengthen your spine, then exhale as you lean gently to one side, creating a stretch along the opposite side of your body.

- Keep both hips grounded on the chair and both feet flat on the floor as you stretch.

- Hold the stretch for several breaths, feeling the lengthening sensation along the side of your body, then repeat on the other side.

4. Seated Chest Opener with Strap:

- Sit tall in your chair with your feet flat on the floor and knees hip-width apart.

- Hold the strap behind your back with both hands, keeping your arms straight and shoulders relaxed.

- Inhale to open your chest and lift your sternum towards the sky, gently pulling the strap apart with your hands.

- Hold the stretch for several breaths, feeling the opening across your chest and shoulders.

5. **Seated Spinal Twist with Strap:**

- Sit tall in your chair with your feet flat on the floor and knees hip-width apart.

- Hold the strap with both hands, extending your arms in front of you at shoulder height.

- Inhale to lengthen your spine, then exhale as you twist gently to one side, bringing the strap across your body.

- Use the strap to deepen the twist, but only go as far as is comfortable for your body.

- Hold the stretch for several breaths, feeling the gentle rotation in your spine, then repeat on the other side.

Chapter 12

Chair Yoga FaQs And Safety Tips

In the Chair Yoga FAQs and Safety Tips section, addressing common concerns and providing solutions is crucial for ensuring a safe and enjoyable practice. Here are some common concerns and their solutions:

1. **Concern:** I'm not flexible enough to do yoga poses.

- **Solution:** Chair yoga is accessible to people of all fitness levels and body types. The poses can be modified to suit your individual needs and abilities. Start with gentle movements and gradually build flexibility over time.

2. **Concern:** I have limited mobility or physical challenges.

- **Solution:** Chair yoga can be adapted to accommodate various physical limitations. Focus on gentle movements, breathwork, and seated poses that feel comfortable and accessible for your body. Use props like bolsters, cushions, and straps to support your practice.

3. **Concern:** I'm worried about falling or losing my balance.

- **Solution:** Practice chair yoga in a safe and stable environment, such as a sturdy chair placed on a non-slip surface. Use the chair for support and balance as needed during standing poses. Move mindfully and within your comfortable range of motion to reduce the risk of falls.

4. **Concern:** I have a medical condition or injury.

- **Solution:** Consult with your healthcare provider before starting any new exercise program, including chair yoga. Inform your yoga instructor about any medical conditions or injuries so they can provide appropriate modifications and ensure your safety during practice.

5. **Concern:** I feel self-conscious practicing yoga in a group setting.

- **Solution:** Chair yoga can be practiced in the comfort of your own home or in a private setting if you prefer. You can also look for chair yoga classes specifically designed for seniors or individuals with mobility challenges, where you'll be practicing with others who have similar needs and experiences.

6. **Concern:** I'm not sure if I'm doing the poses correctly.

- **Solution:** Listen to your body and practice mindfulness during your chair yoga practice. Focus on proper alignment, breathing, and sensation rather than achieving a perfect pose. If you're unsure about a particular pose, ask your yoga instructor for guidance or seek out instructional videos or resources for clarification.

7. **Concern:** I don't have enough time for yoga practice.

- **Solution:** Chair yoga can be practiced in short sessions throughout the day, making it easy to incorporate into your daily routine. Even just a few minutes of gentle movement and relaxation can provide significant benefits for your physical and mental well-being.

8. **Concern:** I experience discomfort or pain during yoga practice.

- **Solution:** Listen to your body and avoid pushing yourself beyond your limits. If a pose causes pain or discomfort, ease out of it or modify it to make it more comfortable. Focus on gentle movements and stretches that feel good for your body.

9. **Concern:** I'm not sure how to breathe properly during yoga practice.

- **Solution:** Practice mindful breathing techniques, such as deep belly breathing or synchronized breath with movement. Your instructor can guide you on proper breathing techniques to enhance relaxation and focus during practice.

10. **Concern:** I feel overwhelmed or anxious during yoga practice.

- **Solution:** Create a calm and soothing atmosphere for your yoga practice by dimming the lights, playing soft music, or lighting candles or incense. Practice mindfulness and relaxation techniques to help quiet the mind and reduce stress and anxiety.

Conclusion

Chair yoga offers numerous benefits for individuals of all ages and abilities, promoting physical health, mental well-being, and relaxation. By addressing common concerns and providing practical solutions, individuals can feel more confident and comfortable practicing chair yoga safely and effectively. Remember to listen to your body, practice mindfulness, and seek guidance from qualified instructors or healthcare professionals as needed. With regular practice and dedication, chair yoga can be a valuable tool for enhancing overall health and quality of life.

Author's Note

To all the wonderful readers who have journeyed through the pages of this book, I extend my heartfelt gratitude and warmest wishes. Your decision to explore the transformative practice of chair yoga speaks volumes about your commitment to self-care, well-being, and personal growth.

As you hold this book in your hands, may you feel a sense of empowerment and possibility, knowing that you have the tools and wisdom within you to cultivate greater balance, comfort, and joy in your life. May the practices and insights shared here serve as a guiding light on your path to health, happiness, and wholeness.

Remember, you are the author of your own story, and each moment is an opportunity to create the life you desire. Whether you're embarking on a new journey of self-discovery or deepening your existing practice, may you find inspiration, support, and encouragement within these pages.

As you integrate the teachings of chair yoga into your daily life, may you experience a profound sense of connection—to yourself, to others, and to the world around you. May you embrace the beauty of each breath, each movement, and each moment, knowing that you are deserving of love, kindness, and compassion.

Thank you for choosing to embark on this journey with me. May your heart be filled with gratitude, your spirit be lifted with joy, and your life be enriched with abundance.

With warmest regards and deepest appreciation,

Christoph Hermann

GET ACCESS TO MY OTHER BOOKS

BY SCANNING THE QR CODE ABOVE